THE COMPLETE KETOGENIC DIET FOR BEGINNERS

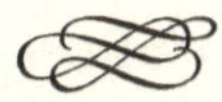

WARAWARAN ROONGRUANGSRI

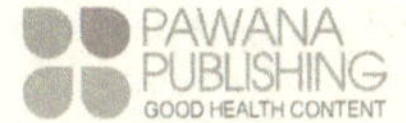

PAWANA PUBLISHING
GOOD HEALTH CONTENT

I love this book! I like introductory to keto and then recipes! It's very simple way to read.

— KRISTIN J. ARNEY

Great guide for beginners, a lot of info, good material to help you reach your goals.

— LUCIA D. HANSEN

This book is easy to follow and explains about how the body works and the recipes are fantastic.

— ANNE J. JOHNSON

INTRODUCTION

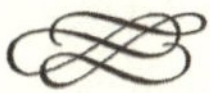

> Some authors describe the ketogenic diet as a low-carbohydrate diet, but this is strictly speaking incorrect. The ketogenic (or keto) diet is in the first instance a high-fat diet that also promotes the consumption of maintenance levels of protein and low levels of carbohydrate.

The keto diet originated as a medical diet that was developed at the Mayo Clinic in the 1920s by **Dr. Russell Morse Wilder** after Woodyatt discovered ketone bodies in the livers of people who ingested no carbohydrates at all.

Over time the keto diet went mainstream, and today the name no longer refers only to diets under medical supervision aimed at the treatment of epilepsy. The various keto regimens made famous by the advocacy of people like Robert Atkins, took the keto diet mainstream, and today the health and benefits of this diet are well accepted and supported by most medical scientists.

The keto diet is not distinguished by limiting carbs, but rather by ingesting enough fat to speed up the metabolism in the absence of large quantities of carbohydrates.

SUGAR: ENEMY ONE

As soon as the body is depleted of carbohydrates, which are stored as energy in the muscles in the form of adenosine triphosphate (ATP), the body reverts to a secondary energy pathway by burning fat for energy.

When the body starts burning fat rather than carbohydrates (carbs) for energy, ketones are formed in the body. Ketones can be measured during the keto diet by measuring the presence of ketones in the urine.

Since the body now burns fat for energy, insulin becomes redundant. Insulin is the hormone that the body employs to store excess energy consumed in the form of carbohydrate, as fat. When there are no carbs to store and when the insulin is at low resting levels. This, along with other changes the body undergoes during ketosis (when the body burns fat for energy in the absence of carbohydrates) makes the keto diet one that not only helps people lose weight and burn fat, but also results in many positive health benefits.

How much of each macronutrient you are allowed to ingest, varies from person to person. As a rule, carbs need to be controlled to remain in ketosis. Some people follow what is known as the induction phase levels of carbs by not exceeding 30 grams per day. Ketosis can however, keep burning fat and speeding up your metabolism, sometimes when you ingest as much as 100g of carbs per day. Use ketostix to measure the ketones in your urine. As long as the ketostix go purple, you are still in ketosis.

Sugar is the chief enemy of ketosis. As long as you do not consume any added sugar, you are set to go.

As long as you ingest enough fats to keep your metabolic flames burning, you are set to go.

GOOD FOR YOU

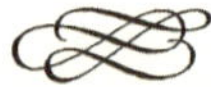

As we already indicated above, the ketogenic diet was developed by researchers at the Mayo Clinic who did not even consider the efficacy of the future keto-diet for weight-loss. After almost a century of research and application, the keto-diet is one of the most researched and most beneficial eating patterns, or diets, in existence. Science has discovered many remarkable properties over the years, and the keto-diet is becoming more popular for it, by the day.

A high carbohydrate diet is a very vague concept. Vegetarians and vegans consume very high amounts of carbs. The modern-day fast food regimen is saturated with enormous levels of carbohydrates. And who can ignore the fact that the latest US Dietary Guidelines advise people to consume between 50-60% carbohydrates in their diet?

Sugars have very little if any health benefits and are on the whole made up of just empty calories, similar to the empty calories alcohol contains, although the alcohol in hard liquors like gin and vodka, whiskey and brandy contain no sugar an can be safely consumed (in moderation) on a keto-diet.

THESE ARE THE BENEFITS

AUTISM

HOW

Some forms of autism respond only on a ketogenic diet. Many autism patients can rely on the ketogenic diet to reduce autistic symptoms and disruptions in their lives.

WHY

This is also related to reduced levels of inflammation and to the increase of certain biological compounds in the brain of keto dieters. One such a substance is adenosine, which is believed to impact the symptoms of autism.

BLOOD SUGAR

HOW

Following the keto diet lowers blood sugar significantly

WHY

Because the body converts fat into energy no sugar is transported through the blood for storage or energy storage, making the production of insulin redundant. This is excellent news for diabetics.

CONCENTRATION

HOW

What a tremendous boost we get from a candy bar or a glass of sugary cool drink. But soon afterward, we need more sugar, more candy and more calories to keep up. If we don't we lose our focus completely

WHY

When we burn fat for energy and produce ketones, there are no spikes and no up and downs. Ketosis burns constant as long as we feed the body enough fat to keep the flames burning. This makes for hyper-concentration

ENERGY
HOW
For many of the same reasons mentioned above. Those on a keto diet have perpetual energy while those who are laden with carbohydrates, sugars and all the water these absorb, will come chuffing along long afterward
WHY
For every gram of carbohydrate ingested and stored in the liver or muscles as glycogen, the body retains another 3 grams of water. This adds bulk and extra weight you have to carry while trying to burn enough carbs for energy. The body cannot burn carbs without storing it first. ATP is produced and stored in the muscles, & glycogen is stored in the liver before the body can "eat its flames." Fat on the other hand, is poured into the bloodstream (straight from the gut) and burn baby burn. The energy is instant and constant.

HUNGER
HOW
No-one on the keto-diet has ever reported that they are hungry, or that they suffer from hunger on a diet. There are no restrictions on your intake. Still hungry, have some more fish, salad, steak or vegetables.
WHY
Since fat is burned for energy and sugar has become redundant for energy production there are no more spikes of hunger, satiety and as blood sugar falls, rising hunger. The fact that is in the bloodstream is consistently burned for energy, so the bodies always have an almost endless supply of

instant fuel. Hunger actually becomes redundant. Also, the hormones that create hunger are influenced by the diet, and switched off.

LONGEVITY

HOW

First off, obesity is toxic and kills. The keto diet brings about rapid weight loss, which already increases longevity. The keto diet has been proven to keep the human brain younger. On the keto diet, your brain's aging is slowed down. A younger brain makes for longer life, ceteris paribus. Since the keto diet makes people more energetic, and prevents bloating and makes the heart work easier (due to a very significant reduction in the amount of water that is retained by the body, in the lungs and in the muscles) as well as due to the rapid weight loss and less fat that surround the inside of the body, around the organs and more, longevity is almost guaranteed.

WHY

Since it has been proven that ketones can pass the blood-brain barrier, this has explained why the ketogenic diet (and the ingestion of MCT Oils) significantly improved the cognitive functioning of those suffering from mild Alzheimer's disease.

Ketones can pass the blood-brain barrier, hence it can provide fuel for the brains of Alzheimer patients whose neurons have lost the ability to use glucose to energize the brain. Consequently the ketones restart the cognition of these patients and provide them with a second chance in life – that is why Alzheimer's are also known as Diabetes Type 3 in some circles.

<u>SKIN CARE</u>

HOW

Following a keto diet has such a massive impact on skin health that it deserves a separate chapter. The keto diet flushes the body with essential fatty acids that the body cannot produce: to have it, is to eat it. If it is not ingested, the body remains deprived of it forever. By consuming lots of fish and nuts, the keto-dieter provides huge amounts of essential fatty acids to the body. Omega-3 fatty acids and omega-6 fatty acids prevent and even heal dry skin, inflammation of the skin that cause peeling and cracking, even scaling and dandruff. Also, keto-dieters consume no trans-fats. Trans-fats are well-known to cause inflammation in the body, and all the symptoms above are in part caused by inflammation.

WHY

The ingestion of MCT Oils present in coconut oil for example, reduces Candida Albicans by almost 25%. This reduces the yeast infections that accompany it, and which causes thrush and skin infections.

So, when the body is flush with essential fatty acids and MCT Oils, the skin holds on to nutrients in a more efficient way and this helps to keep it moist and healthy. The result of this action is a reduced need for the skin to produce oils to compensate for its dryness. Of course, this is the holy grail. The less oil, the less acne, period.

~

THE C-WORD

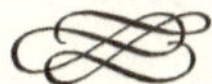

Cancer can be described as the plague of the twenty-first century. Globally, almost ten million people die from it every year. One in six deaths on earth is ascribed to cancer. In the US alone, approximately 1.75 million people will be diagnosed with cancer in 2018, and the outlook is not good. Statistics predict that more than 600,000 of them will not survive their cancer this year.

How ironic then that cancer eats only sugar. It has no use for fat or ketones, and it flourishes in a high-insulin environment. Considering the explosion in the consumption of carbohydrates and refined sugar over the past century, the statistics seem to say that as sugar went up, as did cancer.

To snuff out cancer – to starve it and kill it, we have to avoid sugar and carbohydrates, exactly what the keto diet does. Those on a keto diet ingest no refined sugar and eat very little carbs – something that naturally creates a low-insulin environment, something that naturally prevents cancer from flourishing.

Another way the keto-diet is cancer-unfriendly, is because of its reduced inflammation response. Ketones and ketosis go hand in hand with reduced inflammation throughout the body (as seen above in Chapter 2 for example), and cancer develops in times of inflammation.

Although inflammation is a normal bodily response when healing takes place, prolonged inflammation causes damage to human DNA, and everyone now understands that DNA damage more often than not cause cancer. This is even more marked when considering the fact that individuals who suffer from inflammatory bowel disease for example, have a much higher risk of developing colon cancer.

To come back to eating fat rather than sugar, it follows that a cancer-preventative ketogenic diet will include extreme amounts of fat and virtually no carbohydrates. This way, cancer (might) dies, the patient feels great, and everyone wins!

Numerous studies have indicated the links between cancer and sugar, and between lowered cancer risk and the ketogenic diet, amongst them studies by Siddhartha Mukherjee from University Vagelos College of Physicians and Surgeons from New York City, and Hopkins and Pauli et al. (2018) and many others.

ANTI-CANCER KETOGENIC DIET SUGGESTED FOODS

ANTI-CANCER BENEFITS	EAT OFTEN	EAT NOW & THEN	NEVER EAT
Aids the body's response to repair cancer cells	Cruciferous and leafy green vegetables	Alcoholic beverages like Vodka, whiskey or gin	Beer
Impairs growth of cancer cells	Egg Yolks	Chocolate	Starches (potatoes, fries, bread)
Lowers the insulin levels in the body	Full-fat butter, cheese & cream	Fruits, rarely and then only varieties of berries	Sugar in any form (fruits, candies, cake
Starves the cancer cells	Nuts	Root vegetables like yams	

THE EPILEPSY CONNECTION

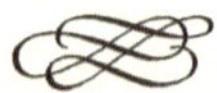

The epilepsy connection has been elucidated already in chapter one above. As explained, the keto diet was developed first and foremost as a treatment for epilepsy. It worked wonders and remained the preferred treatment until the golden era of pharmaceuticals arrived with bottles full of drugs and miles of inserts filled with promises.

> Obviously, when the anti-seizure drugs work, it is much preferred as a treatment and makes the whole ketogenic diet redundant. One has to keep in mind that the original ketogenic diet was a strictly supervised medical nutritional treatment offered by a whole team of specialists and nutritionists.

Epilepsy is a serious neurological condition that has many causes and few cures. Epilepsy can be acquired by infection, stroke or traumatic brain injuries, but it can also be genetic, which is the cause in the majority of cases. Irrespective of the causes of epilepsy, the symptoms can be quite debilitating. Patients suffer from convulsions or seizures, or both, and due to the unpredictability and sudden onset of the same, these "attacks" are often suffered in public. The symptoms, which lead to the condition being called falling-sickness amongst other names, still lead to some social stigma, and may isolate and socially impair sufferers. It is not an insignificant condition, and as such, those suffering from it without the relief obtained from anti-seizure medications, are severely impaired.

For the children who live with persistent seizures despite taking medications the keto diet offers the best hope. Peer-reviewed studies indicate that these children obtain great relief from their seizures by just eating keto. A significant number of these children experience up to a ninety percent reduction of symptoms.

When studies compared the efficacy of the keto diet with seizure medications, the surprising result showed that three-quarters of all the subjects in the keto-group experienced reduced seizures.

〜

THE SILENT KILLER

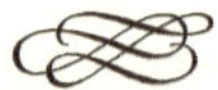

Blood pressure kills. It is as simple as that. It goes hand in hand with aging, obesity and diet. It becomes a silent killer for those who remain symptom-free and have no inclination to seek treatment because they feel great.

Those who suffer from both high blood pressure and diabetes, double their risk of early death. The third major risk factor is cholesterol. Those who suffer from all three, have real problems.

Physicians treat high blood pressure with medications. Proper medication can have a wonderful effect on high blood pressure and can be a real lifesaver. For many, blood pressure medication, although it does what it is supposed to, cause unpleasant side-effects that sometimes cause more distress than the original symptoms. This population is at risk because they often have greater motivation not to take their medicine.

As mentioned above, the consumption of carbohydrates leads to very high water retention. When the body bloats and retains water, this has a very negative impact on blood pressure.

The same goes for obesity. The bigger you become, as a general rule, the harder your heart works, and for most people, this is concomitant with rising blood pressure.

What is more, the more bloated or the more obese you become, the lower your energy levels drop, and this leads to inactivity. There is a common saying in biology: inactivity kills. This becomes a vicious circle. More food, more blood pressure, more fat, more sugar, less activity, and more fat, more blood pressure, and so on.

During peer-reviewed double-blind studies, 50% of the group who followed a ketogenic diet showed a significant decrease in blood pressure, while the low-fat diet group, who lost similar amounts of weight, showed a 50% lower reduction in blood pressure. The researchers concluded that a reduction in carbohydrates was a significant indicator in the reduction of blood pressure.

It is precautious for those who follow the ketogenic diet to add as many foods high in potassium to their diets as they can. Potassium is well known as the element that regulates blood pressure in the body. If taken in large enough quantities (up to 5,000 mg per day), it can reduce blood pressure significantly. Several foods included in the ketogenic diet contain high amounts of potassium:

- Asparagus
- Avocado
- Broccoli
- Brussel Sprouts
- Spinach
- Tomatoes
- Zucchini

Some foods high in potassium are expressly **NOT** allowed on the ketogenic diet. Some of these are:

- Bananas
- Coconut Water
- Dried Apricots
- Pomegranate
- Sweet Potato
- White Beans

SO WHAT CAN I EAT WHEN I DO THE KETO?

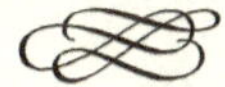

YES AND NO. THE TRUTH ABOUT GOING KETO. It is very important to understand something that seems counterintuitive before you start on the keto diet for the first time.

- **Yes**, the ketogenic diet is a high fat diet.
- **No**, the ketogenic diet does not increase cholesterol levels.
- **Yes**, the ketogenic diet will actually decrease your bad cholesterol, increase your good cholesterol, and improve your cholesterol profile.
- **No**, we do not get fat by eating fat – it is a false assumption that leads to the carb-crazy low-fat high-carb diets of the period between 1990 and 2010. It has been thoroughly discredited. It is not fat that makes you fat. It is not only calories that make you fat.

ON THE KETOGENIC DIET, you can eat a lot more calories –

and lose weight. And, on the ketogenic diet, you can lean in and eat all your favorite fatty treats. Counterintuitively, the more fat you eat, the more weight you lose. It's that simple.

The ketogenic diet is an unprocessed food diet. And it is a sugar-avoidant diet. Carbohydrates, the good ones, are allowed, and some vegetables are free goods that can be consumed at will, regardless of quantity. Fat is needed as a fuel, and this is utilized and converted into energy by the body, while flushing the system with essential fatty acids your body cannot produce for itself.

The ketogenic diet is a healthy diet – in fact, it is the number one "health diet" in the world. Just do it, and you'll never look back.

YES-FOODS AND NO-FOODS FOR THE KETOGENIC DIET

SEAFOOD

EXAMPLES

Salmon and sardines, tuna and squid, mussels and prawns, clams, halibut and oysters, crabs and lobster, flounder, herring, sole, trout and cod.

TIPS

Most of these foods can be eaten in almost unlimited amounts as often as possible. Seafood is healthy and so beneficial, your body will just flourish.

COMMENTS

Try to eat seafood at least once a day if you can afford it. More is better.

NO-FOODS

Seafood that is coated in flour and cereal or any other carb-rich foods. And no, regrettably fries are not seafood!

<u>VEGETABLES</u>

EXAMPLES

Olives, Radishes, Spinach, Lettuce, Mushrooms, Celery, Spinach, Broccoli, Avocado, Onions, Cucumber, Asparagus, Peppers, Tomatoes, Brussel Sprouts, Spaghetti Squash, Pumpkin, Green Beans

TIPS

Again, almost all of these vegetables can be eaten in virtually unlimited quantities.

COMMENTS

Understand that keto vegetables exclude all starches.

NO-FOODS

Carrots, Peas, Sweet Potatoes, Potatoes, Beetroot, Rice, Beans (only green beans are allowed), no grains or cereals. None.

<u>DAIRY PRODUCTS</u>

EXAMPLES

Butter, Cheddar, Gouda, Cream Cheese, Swiss, Feta, Mozzarella, Blue Cheese and heavy, whipping and pouring cream.

TIPS

These cheeses are allowed on the ketogenic diet. Limit cheese to 4 or 5 oz. per day.

COMMENTS

Do not overdo the cheeses and the butter. Cheese contains about 1 gram of carbs per oz. so limit your intake accordingly. Cheeses not listed should be avoided.

NO-FOODS

No milk or yogurt. Both are sugar-rich and will hinder ketosis.

MEAT & POULTRY
EXAMPLES
Beef, Lamb, Pork, Venison, Bacon, Ham, Chicken, Duck, Ostrich, Turkey, Goose, Pheasant
TIPS
Cut and enjoy. Get enough protein to satisfy your cravings. Do not cut off the fat.
COMMENTS
Do not overdo it. Excess protein can be converted into sugar in the body, so make sure that you ingest enough fatty cuts. Limit bacon and ham that are cured using sugar, and avoid foods that contain high nitrates.
NO-FOODS
Recipes that contain sugar or coatings that contain flour or carbs, or cured meats containing sugar. Be carb-savvy and read food labels.

EGGS
EXAMPLES
Soft or hard, boiled, poached, scrambled or fried in butter, omelet or deviled
TIPS
This is nature's perfect food. Do not eat egg whites only – always eat the yolks too.
COMMENTS
Eggs are a perfect protein and it's versatile so you can combine it with cheese, butter and vegetables to create delicious meals.

OILS & FATS
EXAMPLES
Butter, Mayonnaise (products with no added sugars),

Olive oil, Canola, Walnut, Grape Seed, Sesame, Coconut Oil

TIPS

Great way to add fats to the diet. It is entirely carb free. Do not overheat oils and do not cook with sesame or walnut oil – use for salads only.

COMMENTS

Coconut Oil is a superfood that contains MCT Oils.

NO-FOODS

No form of trans fats. No food that has trans fats in it, can be eaten. No margarine products.

FRUITS

EXAMPLES

Berries: Strawberries, blackberries, blueberries and mulberries

TIPS

To quote Dr. Robert Atkins: "Since when does fruit have such a good reputation."

COMMENTS

Fruits are overrated. They are nature's way to store sugar. Avoid. If you eat berries, limit it. Do not overindulge.

NO-FOODS

Avoid all fruits except berries. It is advisable to only start eating berries after six months when you have overcome all your carb-cravings and reached your goal weight.

NUTS

EXAMPLES

Pecans, Macadamia and Brazil

TIPS

These nuts can be eaten in almost unlimited quantities on the keto diet.

COMMENTS

Eat Hazelnuts, Walnuts and Almonds in great moderation.

NO-FOODS

Avoid peanuts, cashews and pistachio nuts.

ALCOHOL

EXAMPLES

Hard Liquor. Whisky, Gin, Vodka, Tequila, Vodka

TIPS

Alcohol contains as much calories as pure fat, empty calories, but is contains zero carbs and can be consumed.

COMMENTS

Moderation

NO-FOODS

No wine, cocktails or coolers, and no beer or ciders.

SUGAR

EXAMPLES

None. Zero. Zilch. Use artificial Sweeteners at will. Do not worry about "sugar alcohols, they actually cancel out the carbs in a food. You can subtract sugar alcohols and fibre from the carb count to calculate the net carb content of a food.

TIPS

Sugar will stop ketosis dead in its tracks.

COMMENTS

Don't.

NO-FOODS

All Sugars. All of them!

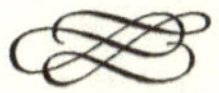

KETOGENIC DIET IS NOT A LOW-CARB DIET

As explained above, the ketogenic diet is not a low-carb diet – it is high fat, medium protein and low carb diet. Describing the keto diet as low-carb is fundamentally erroneous. On a real low-carb diet, you can consume pure sugar, or candy bars every day as long as you keep your carbohydrate intake low. When mainstream nutrition describes low-carbs, they mean anything below fifty percent of daily intake.

In essence, low-carb is a diet that restricts carbohydrates without restricting specific types of carbohydrates. Low-carb does not restrict the use of honey for example, a delicious foodstuff that is absolutely disallowed on any ketogenic menu.

To be clear, the ketogenic diet is a diet that restricts carbohydrates, yes – but only some carbohydrates. Honey is an absolute no, but pumpkin is a yes. It is just a misnomer to confuse the ketogenic with low-carb regimens.

THE PALEO DIET IS NOT KETOGENIC, BUT IT CAN BE

Another case in point – the paleo diet might be a wonderful diet that is followed with great fanfare by millions, but the paleo is by no means a ketogenic diet. A paleo diet can become ketogenic, if the rules of the ketogenic, the philosophy, are incorporated into the paleo regimen. Many such diets do the rounds, but then the paleo is actually just a restricted ketogenic diet.

Paleo adherents eat fruit for example, in the way they anticipate our forefathers did when they roamed the plains and lived wild and free. On the ketogenic diet, we severely restrict fruits, even those our forebears might have consumed in abundance. Sugar for the ketogenic adherent, is public enemy number one.

The ketogenic diet is all about ketosis, and you have to understand ketosis to be able to follow the ketogenic diet successfully. Although we discussed ketosis above in some detail, some more detail will suffice.

FAT IS PERFECT ENERGY

The body stores all its excess energy in the form of fat, a substance that can be very quickly changed back into pure energy in the form of fatty acids and glycerol. When the body stops using carbohydrates as a primary source of fuel, the body simply starts using its reserve energy by converting it in this way.

FAT IS CRUCIAL IF YOU WANT TO STAY ALIVE

Keep in mind that fat is a very important substance for human health.

VITAMINS AND MACRONUTRIENTS

It does not only store and provides energy; it also stores micronutrients like vitamins that are fat-soluble. Fat-soluble micronutrients can only be stored and distributed through the body by fats. No other distribution is possible.

TEMPERATURE AND IMMUNE SYSTEM

Fat also controls body temperature and healthy cell functioning. It is crucial for the functioning of the immune system as well. The body rids itself of toxins by filtering it "through" fats and depositing it in the fat stores before removing it from the body.

LIPOLYSIS & KETOSIS

During lipolysis the body switches to using fat rather than sugar as an energy source. A ketosis is a form of lipolysis and when the body is starved off carbohydrates, lipolysis produces ketones as a by-product.

It takes the body an average of 48-hours to switch from using sugar (carbohydrates) for energy to lipolysis (ketosis). That is why it is so important not to cheat when you are on the ketogenic diet. If you quickly dive into a cheeseburger and fries, washed down with a shake, just as a treat or cheat when doing the keto, ketosis will screech to a halt, and you will only get the ketones flowing and get back into ketosis after another 48-hours. It is not worth it.

Since fat is a far superior and much faster source of fuel for the body (the body was designed to store energy as fat, and not as sugar - the perfect form of energy that can be converted by the body into energy almost instantly) ketosis feels like a turbo boost for most people.

The energy produced is intense, focused and constant.

There are no signs of peaks and valleys. Morning, noon or night, you will either be supercharged or asleep in bed. And because the energy flow is so constant and so readily available, hunger becomes a thing of the past. The body no longer has to signal you to get food soon, our supply is running low. The supply now becomes unlimited. The only requirement is to keep the fire burning. Keep the flame alive by making absolutely sure that you ingest enough fat every day and during the day, to kick-start the fat-generator built into your body.

INTERMITTENT FASTING IS AN EATING PATTERN, NOT A DIET

Many people also misunderstand the differences between intermittent fasting and the ketogenic diet. Again, these are things apart, but they can be incorporated. Hence, some ketogenic dieters incorporate a form of intermittent fasting, while some intermittent fasters incorporate ketogenic principles into their fasting method.

I digress – intermittent fasting is not a diet. It is an eating pattern. It does not prescribe what should be eaten, only when it should be eaten. This means that a vegan on an 80% carbohydrate diet can follow the eating pattern, by fasting for, say, 18 hours every day, and eating for only six hours.

No doubt, many people experience huge benefits from this, and from the ketogenic community, we wish them well. When you want to incorporate intermittent fasting into your ketogenic diet, that is, if you want to follow the ketogenic diet but also want to follow the intermittent eating pattern, just do it.

However, some issues need clarification. Intermittent fasting aficionados often proclaim the benefits of ketosis as a basis for their claims. Most of them however, is just wrong.

Ketosis takes fasting of 48-hours – that is, a period of 48 carbohydrate free hours before it kicks in. It is highly unlikely, and there is no evidence available, that the body will go into lipolysis – or ketosis – within eighteen hours after the start of a fast.

MCT OILS

True enough, by adding so-called bulletproof coffees infused with pure MCT Oils, this process has been proven to become more rapid, and MCT Oils can greatly benefit those who use it.

Those who streamline the ketogenic diet by adding intermittent fasting will turbocharge their turbocharged weight loss program. The longer the body remains in ketosis without ingesting any calories, logically, the more weight will be lost, faster. However, it is strongly advised that you add MCT Oils to coffee or even, as some pundits advise, some butter to your coffee just to keep the flames burning hot and keep the ketosis "machine" running smoothly.

The basic way to add the intermittent fasting pattern to the ketogenic diet is to just skip breakfast and only pop a quick bulletproof MCT Oil infused morning coffee. Wait eighteen hours after your last meal of the previous day, before eating your first meal. It is not hard to do on the ketogenic diet at all. And the benefits are legion. The only requirement is that you attempt to keep a rigid schedule. Fast daily, but break your fast exactly at the same time every day. The body flourishes when rigid routines are followed. This eliminates shock from your system.

~

BEGINNING IS THE HARDEST PART

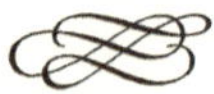

*E*ASE INTO IT

There are as many philosophies about how one should start as there are pundits. The way I approach it, is to ease into the new lifestyle. I actually advise that proponents gain a few pounds over the last week or two before digging in. Go out and overdue (do it over, don't overdo) your favorite unhealthy treats a bit. Have a few extra slices of cake and eat a few burgers with fries. And gain a pound or two. It is easier to start on the ketogenic diet if you can truly say "I have had it. I am so over sugar. Or fries."

It is also very easy to drop off the pound or two gained over the last month before you start on the keto. It's as if the last month's fat stores only rented space with the option to buy, when you sold off space to the ketogenic diet.

COMMIT

When you are ready, because you are sick of eating all those white and empty carbs, commit to a date, and now prepare your tools. This will now be easier because you overindulged a bit on your favorite foods. You will be able to circumvent the omnipresent sense of loss many experiences when they say goodbye for now to the comfort foods that delivered them in voluptuous form at the front door of the ketogenic diet.

WEIGH YOURSELF – AND WRITE IT DOWN!

Weigh yourself. This is so important, because, believe it or not, when the pounds start melting of as quick as it does on the keto diet, you will actually suffer disbelief and start rationalizing that you actually were not that fat. You have to write your weight down, or will suffer from denial when the great melting begins.

REMOVE YOURSELF FROM TEMPTATION

Clear your home of as many keto-unfriendly foods as you can. This is easy enough if you live alone, or if you are joined by your spouse, but is can be quite tricky if your family refuses to support you. If the fridge remains filled with ice cream and pies, the keto can become a test of your perseverance over the first three weeks or so.

FAMILY AND FRIENDS

If your family is planning to "laugh" at you while they down shake and crunchy fries, try to negotiate a truce: try to "buy them off" to arrange a food free zone for the first three or four weeks. After the first month, you will be immune against cravings. You will see food in a new way: almost as an observer. You will no longer be obsessed with nice comfortable foods to down your sorrows in. You will actually become the person that forgets to eat or eats only when they are hungry, not because it is lunchtime. So, do the truce if you can.

OLD FAVORITES

Your favorite meals do not have to be exterminated from your mind. Once you passed the dangerous first three weeks, your world can open to all the available substitute products on the market today. On the keto diet you can now buy chocolate and candy bars (think Atkins for example), ice cream and pancakes, pretty much anything you can dream off, in a delicious zero carb ketogenic form.

But, alas, try to avoid these luxuries during the first month. After the first, you will no longer be vulnerable to weaknesses of the flesh. You will rule the food, not the other way around.

THE COLOR PURPLE: KETOSTIX

Always monitor your ketones. Buy ketostix, or an electronic monitor, and measure your ketone level during the day – in the beginning – as often as possible. Whenever the strip turns purple, you are in the zone. Purple equals losing fat right now.

By monitoring this, you will quickly learn how to keep feeding the body enough fats during the day to keep the purple as dark as possible, and you will learn to regret deviations and cheats when you are back to plain yellow – and out of ketosis. Just remember that you have to measure 'your failure' after cheats long enough after the event. Only urine produced after the fact will be free from ketones, and expose your lack of ketosis.

DRINK WATER OR DIE

Hydration is probably the most important thing to keep in mind on the keto diet. Remember, your body stops retaining water per carb ingested, so you will naturally lose such a lot of water that you will feel thinner even before starting to lose weight. But you will also feel warmer, and you might suffer from a sense of dry mouth or even a sense of tiredness pretty soon if you do not hydrate properly.

Now that you are carb free, the water will basically run right through you. So you have to drink water and then some. Drink until you need to urinate, and then replenish your stores with 50% more than you lose through urination, every time, around the clock. You have to drink to survive and to melt. And then some.

GOING SOCIAL IS NOT THAT HARD

Many books and pundits make a big deal of eating out, social events and celebrations. We do not. Once you are in ketosis, you develop a sense of purpose and satiety that will normally safeguard you from temptation. Carry some keto-genic candy bars, some nuts and a beverage of your choice, as well as some sweetener with you at all times. When drinks are poured, pour your own if no one catered for your prefer-ence. If you are having coffee, pop out your own sweetener and even pocket creamies, when required. And when dessert is carried in, have a chocolate bar with a handful of salty nuts. You will not be tempted by anything.

CHEATER EATER

From time to time you will ingest "forbidden foods" by accident. Do not fret. It won't kill you, it will only educate you. Just make very sure that you order and purchase and eat only suitable foods wherever you go. Often servers will just lie about the recipes. As soon as you tell them that you cannot have anything with flour in it, for example – 'because I will die if I do' they quickly confess and provide you with the truth.

RUN-FROM PEOPLE

Just remember, those people around you that are constantly trying to get you to 'just have one, you also have a right to enjoy yourself' and so on, are not really your friends. They are run from people who actively encourage you to fail. Explain it to your friends and family once, and then demand support after that.

EXERCISE IS GOOD BUT NOT REQUIRED

It is unimportant from a weight-loss point of view to exercising while you are on the ketogenic diet. You will lose massive amounts of fat even if you are the ultimate couch potato. If you are severely obese or overweight, I would advise that you wait for as long as it takes you to become more comfortable physically and less self-conscious.

ABUNDANT ENERGY

Once you become infused with unlimited keto-energy, things will naturally change. You will simply want to get up, out & about. Your energy levels will be concomitant with a faster and more efficient metabolism and any signs of pre-diabetes will disappear. Now is the time to seize the day. Walk, run, swim, gym – do it all, or do only one. Exercise is only harmful when you are seriously ill.

HOW LONG ON KETO? HOW LONG IS A PIECE OF ROPE?

Asking how long you should stay on the ketogenic diet is the wrong question, quite frankly. Some people only do the keto diet to lose a few pounds, and then they revert to their old lifestyle. Remember, the keto diet is more of a lifestyle than a diet. Going back to the diet that made you fat and slow, is like going out to try and get the flu virus back after you were cured.

Some people stay on the ketogenic diet for the rest of their lives. The ketogenic diet is not a small thing. It has dimensions and various phases that you can develop to adapt to your changing requirements. This book covers the first phase. There are many more that can be followed up by future publications.

PLEASE COME BACK SOON

For those who lost the weight, but do not feel at home on the keto diet, that is perfectly alright too. Eat the fat, lose the weight. Then leave. No problem. Just come back if you get fat and fatigued again.

It is up to every individual, there are no minimums or maximums. Keep going as long as you feel that you benefit. Come back if you feel you need to. It is a way of life to come and go, too.

~

7 DAY MEAL PLAN AND RECIPES FOR KETO DIET

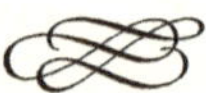

*E*njoy the top keto recipes, with simple instructions

DAY 1

Breakfast: Mini Crustless Quiches

Ingredients

- Eggs 14 large
- Diced soppressata salami ⅔ cup
- Diced tomatoes 3 plum
- Diced sweet onion ⅓ cup
- Shredded mozzarella cheese ⅔ cup
- Shredded pepper jack cheese ⅓ cup
- Sliced pickled jalapenos ⅓ cup
- Heavy cream ⅓ cup

Instructions

1. Preheat the oven to 325°F
2. Grease a 15"×11" muffin tin

3. Add all of ingredients together in a mixing bowl
4. Season with salt & pepper
5. Now whisk the ingredients in the mixing bowl thoroughly
6. Pour the batter equally into the muffin tin (12 portions)
7. Bake for 25 minutes or until golden brown
8. Serves 12
9. Store in fridge and reheat before serving

Lunch: Ham and Cheddar Wraps
Ingredients

- Deli ham 2 oz.
- Shredded cheddar 2 oz.
- Mayonnaise 2 tbsp
- Low carb wrap 1 wrap
- Pickles or jalapenos to taste
- Salt, pepper to taste

Instructions

1. Spread mayonnaise onto a low-carb wrap
2. Now add shredded cheddar cheese and ham slices
3. Add jalapeños or pickles according to taste
4. Roll the wrap up tightly

DINNER: Chicken and Mushrooms
Ingredients

- Chicken breast 6 oz.
- Butter 2 tbsp

- Heavy cream ¼ cup
- White mushrooms 8 oz.
- Spinach 1 handful
- Water ¼ cup
- Fresh lemon juice 1 tsp
- Salt, pepper to taste

Instructions

1. Place a pan on medium heat
2. Add chicken and then cook until it is almost done
3. Remove from the pan and plate it to cool down
4. Add some butter into the same pan and then add the mushrooms
5. Over medium heat, cook the mushrooms until they shrink and start to crisp up
6. Then add water, lemon juice and heavy cream and stir well
7. Cook until the sauce thickens
8. Season the sauce with salt & pepper
9. Now return the chicken back into the sauce and cook until warm

DAY 2

Breakfast: Cheese Roll

Ingredients

- Sliced cheddar cheese 8 oz.
- Butter 2 oz.

Instructions

1. Place cheese slices on a large cutting board

2. Slice butter with a cheese slicer into very thin slices
3. Cover every cheese slice with a butter slice and roll up
4. Serve as a snack

LUNCH: Caprese Omelet

Ingredients

- Sliced mozzarella cheese 5 oz.
- Fresh basil or dried basil 1 tbsp
- Sliced tomatoes 3 oz.
- Olive oil 2 tbsp
- Eggs 2 large

Instructions

1. Add the eggs into a mixing bowl
2. Add salt & pepper to taste
3. Whisk very well with a fork
4. When the egg mix is well combined, add basil and stir
5. Now slice the tomatoes and cheese
6. Using a large pan over medium heat, add some oil and then add the tomato slices
7. Fry tomatoes for a few minutes until done
8. Into the same pan, pour the egg mix over the fried tomatoes
9. Wait until the egg mix firms up slightly, then add the mozzarella cheese
10. Lower the heat and wait for the omelet to set
11. Serve hot

DINNER: Meat Pie

Ingredients

- Ground beef or ground lamb 20 oz.
- Butter or olive oil 2 tbsp
- Finely chopped garlic clove 1 tbsp
- Finely chopped yellow onion ½ large
- Dried oregano or dried basil 1 tbsp
- Tomato paste 4 tbsp
- Water ½ cup

Instructions

1. Preheat the oven to 350°F
2. In a saucepan over medium heat, add some butter and garlic, and then add the onions
3. Fry onion for a few minutes until translucent
4. When the onions are translucent, add the ground beef and keep on frying
5. Add oregano and add salt & pepper
6. Add tomato paste (or pesto/jar) and add some water
7. Lower the heat, and then simmer for at least 20 minutes
8. In the meantime, add all the dough ingredients in a food processor
9. Mix it until turns into a ball
10. Place piece of round parchment paper in a well-greased springform pan
11. Spread the dough in the pan and fold it up along the sides
12. Pre bake the crust in the oven for 15 minutes

13. Remove the crust from the oven
14. Remove the saucepan from the heat ad spoon the meat into the crust
15. Mix the cottage cheese and the shredded cheddar cheese
16. Layer the cheese over the top of the meat in the crust
17. Bake for 30 minutes or until golden brown
18. Serve with fresh green salad and dressing of choice

DAY 3

Breakfast: Chocolate Pancakes with Blueberry Butter
Ingredients

- Eggs 4 large
- Frozen wild blueberries 3 tbsp
- Chocolate Collagen Protein 1 scoop
- Coconut oil 3 tbsp
- Coconut flour ¼ scant cup
- Baking soda ½ tbsp
- Kerry Gold butter for cooking 1 tbsp
- Kerry Gold butter 2 tbsp

Instructions

1. Place the large iron skillet over medium heat
2. In the mixing bowl, add the eggs and MCT Oil and whisk well. Add the coconut flour, protein powder and baking soda as well as a pinch of salt
3. Mix until smooth and creamy
4. Now add a tablespoon of butter to the skillet
5. Add ⅔ of a cup of batter into the skillet and cook on medium heat for 4 minutes before turning

6. Press down on the pancake and to ensure that the middle cooks through
7. Flip again before removing from heat
8. In a small sauce-pot add the blueberries
9. Cook it on medium heat until they thaw and start to simmer
10. Now add the butter and mix and mash until a soft smooth mix forms
11. Serve your pancakes and spoon the buttery blueberry mix all over them

LUNCH: Turkey Sausage Frittata

Ingredients

- Egg 12 large
- Ground breakfast sausage, turkey 12 oz.
- Shredded cheddar cheese 2 oz.
- Lactose free sour cream 1 cup
- Pink Himalayan salt 1 tbsp
- Bell peppers 2 oz
- Black pepper 1 tbsp
- Kerry Gold butter 2 tbsp

Instructions

1. Preheat the oven to 350°F
2. Add all the eggs to a blender and add the sour cream, salt & pepper and blend on high for 30-seconds
3. Set the mix aside
4. Over medium heat, place a large skillet and add butter when sizzling hot

5. Add the bell peppers, sliced into strips into the skillet.
6. Sauté the peppers for six minutes (or until brown and tender)
7. Now remove the peppers from the skillet
8. Add the turkey sausage to the skillet and stir to break it up evenly
9. Fry for 8 minutes or until brown
10. Flatten the turkey on the bottom of the skillet
11. Place the peppers over the sausage, as evenly as possible
12. Pour the egg mix over the peppers and sausage
13. Now place the skillet into the preheated oven and bake for 30 minutes.
14. Add cheese by sprinkling it over the frittata as soon as you take it from the oven

DINNER: Delicious Low Carb Keto Meatloaf

Ingredients

- Eggs 2 large
- Ground beef 2 pounds
- Black pepper 1 tbsp
- Nutritional Yeast ¼ cup
- Avocado oil 1 tbsp
- Garlic 4 cloves
- Lemon zest 1 tbsp
- Chopped parsley ¼ cup
- Chopped fresh oregano ¼ cup
- Pink Himalayan salt ½ tbsp

Instructions

1. Preheat the oven to 400°F
2. In the large mixing bowl, add ground beef, salt, black pepper and the yeast
3. Add the eggs, oil, lemon, herbs and garlic to a blender and blend until the eggs form a mousse and the ingredients are minced and mixed
4. Add the egg blend to the beef and mix well to combine
5. Add the beef-egg mix into a small 8"×4" loaf pan
6. Smooth the mix and flatten it out
7. Place into an oven and bake for 50 minutes or until golden brown
8. Remove the loaf pan from the oven
9. Over the sink, turn the loaf pan over carefully and drain the fluid from it
10. Let a meatloaf cool for 10 minutes before slicing
11. Garnish with lemon and serve

DAY 4

Breakfast: Chocolate Peanut Butter Muffins

Ingredients

- Eggs 2 large
- SF chocolate chips ½ cup
- almond flour 1 cup
- erythritol ½ cup
- baking powder 1 tbsp
- peanut butter ⅓ cup
- almond milk ⅓ cup
- salt 1 pinch

Instructions

1. Combine all of dry ingredients (except the chocolate chips) into a large mixing bowl and stir well
2. Add the peanut butter and almond milk and stir until well-combined
3. Add one egg at a time to the mix, folding each one in fully
4. Then fold in the chocolate chips
5. Spray the muffin tin with cook & spray and add the batter
6. Bake for 15 minutes at 350°F
7. Six muffins serves three

LUNCH: Cheddar Chicken and Broccoli Casserole
Ingredients

- Crushed pork rinds 1 oz
- Shredded chicken breast, 20 oz.
- Shredded cheddar cheese 1 cup
- Broccoli florets 2 cups
- Sour cream ½ cup
- Heavy cream ½ cup
- Olive oil 2 tbsp
- Salt, pepper to taste
- Oregano 1 tsp

Instructions

1. Preheat the oven to 450°F
2. In a mixing bowl, combine the chicken, broccoli florets, olive oil and sour cream and stir well
3. Grease a 8"×11" baking dish

4. Spoon the mix evenly into the baking dish
5. Now drizzle the heavy cream over the ingredients of the baking dish
6. Season with salt & pepper and oregano
7. Top the dish with cheddar cheese and top the cheese with the crushed pork rinds
8. Bake for 25 minutes until golden brown

DINNER: Shrimp and Mushroom Zoodles

Ingredients

- Parmesan cheese 2 tbsp
- Peeled large shrimp 6 oz.
- Sliced white mushrooms 8 oz.
- Zucchini 1 large
- Marinara sauce ¼ cup
- Olive oil 1 tbsp
- Butter 1 tbsp
- Salt, pepper to taste

Instructions

1. In the large pan, over medium heat, heat the olive oil
2. Add the mushrooms and fry until most of the oil is absorbed
3. Now add butter and cook the mushrooms until golden brown
4. Add the shrimps and cook for approximately 4 minutes on each side
5. Using a spiralizer, make the zoodles while the shrimp cooks

6. When the shrimps are cooked through and pink, add the zoodles and toss for about 2 minutes
7. When done, add the marinara sauce and season with salt & pepper

DAY 5

Breakfast: Baked Bacon Omelet

Ingredients

- Eggs 4 large
- Bacon cut in cubes 5 oz.
- Butter 3 oz.
- Fresh spinach 2 oz.
- Finely chopped fresh chives 1 tbsp
- Salt and pepper to taste

Instructions

1. Preheat the oven to 400°F
2. Grease a baking dish with butter
3. In a saucepan, over medium heat, add a remaining butter and fry the bacon and spinach
4. In the mixing bowl, add eggs and whisk well
5. Add the bacon, spinach and the remaining butter from the pan to the egg mix
6. Add the chives and salt & pepper to taste
7. Pour the egg mix into the baking dish and bake for 20 minutes or until golden brown
8. Remove from an oven and allow it to cool down before serving

LUNCH: Smoked Salmon Plate
Ingredients

- Smoked salmon ¾ lb
- Baby spinach 2 oz.
- Mayonnaise 1 cup
- Olive oil 1 tbsp
- Lime (optional) ½
- Salt, pepper to taste

Instructions

1. Plate the salmon with spinach and a wedge of lime
2. Add a dollop of mayonnaise
3. Drizzle an olive oil over the spinach, and season with salt & pepper

DINNER: Asian Cabbage Stir-fry
Ingredients

- Ground beef 20 oz.
- Green cabbage 25 oz.
- Butter 5 oz.
- Sesame oil 1 tbsp
- salt 1 tsp
- Onion powder 1 tsp
- Finely chopped fresh ginger 1 tbsp
- Ground black pepper ¼ tsp
- White wine vinegar 1 tbsp
- Garlic 2 cloves
- Sliced callions 3
- Chili flakes 1 tsp

- Wasabi mayonnaise: Mayonnaise 1 cup and Wasabi paste 1 tbsp

Instructions

1. Shred a cabbage finely using a food processor (or sharp knife)
2. In a wok over medium heat, add 90g of butter
3. When a butter starts to sizzle, add a cabbage and fry until soft
4. Add spices and vinegar and fry for a while longer but remove before the cabbage turns brown
5. Spoon the cabbage into a bowl
6. In the same frying pan, on the medium heat, melt the rest of the butter
7. Add garlic, ginger and chili flakes and sauté for a minute or two
8. Now add the ground meat and brown until thoroughly cooked
9. When most of the liquids have evaporated, lower the heat
10. Add scallions and cabbage and stir until evenly warm
11. Add salt & pepper to taste
12. Top the dish with sesame oil before serving
13. Mix the wasabi with mayonnaise in small amounts until the taste satisfies.
14. Serve the stir fry with a dollop of wasabi mayonnaise

DAY 6

Breakfast: Acai Almond Butter Smoothie
Ingredients

- Unsweetened Acai puree 1,100 g Pack
- Unsweetened almond milk ¾ cup
- Collagen or protein powder 3 tbsp
- Avocado ¼
- Almond butter 1 tbsp
- Coconut oil 1 tbsp
- Vanilla extract ½ tsp
- Liquid stevia 2 drops

Instructions

1. Run the packaged acai puree under lukewarm water until soft enough to break into smaller pieces
2. Now add 100g of acai puree to a blender
3. Add all remaining ingredients into the blender, and blend until creamy and smooth
4. Add more ice or water according to taste
5. Drizzle almond butter on the inside of the glass
6. Serve immediately

LUNCH: **Low Carb Lasagna**

Ingredients

- Spicy Italian sausage ½ lb
- Ricotta cheese 15 oz.
- Butter, ghee, coconut oil, or lard 1 tbsp
- Egg 1 large
- Mozzarella cheese 1 ½ cup
- Parmesan cheese 1/3 cup
- Coconut flour 2 tbsp
- Salt 1 ½ tbsp

- Pepper ½ tbsp
- Garlic powder 1 tbsp
- Finely chopped clove garlic 1 large
- Zucchini's (sliced long ways to 1/4" pieces) 4 large
- Rao's marinara sauce 16 oz.
- Mixed Italian herb seasoning 1 tbsp
- Red pepper flake ½ tbsp
- Basil ¼ cup

Instructions

1. Slice the zucchini thinly and sprinkle with sea salt
2. Place the zucchini on a paper towel for 30 minutes
3. After 30 minutes, wring the last of the moisture from the zucchini one more time using a paper towel
4. In the large skillet, over a medium high heat, add one tablespoon of butter
5. When the butter sizzles, crumble in the Italian sausage
6. When it done, remove from heat and allow meat to cool
7. Preheat the oven to 375°F
8. Coat a 9"×9" baking dish with cook & spray
9. In a mixing bowl, add ricotta cheese about 1 cup of mozzarella cheese, 2 tablespoons of parmesan cheese, 1 egg, coconut flour, salt & pepper, garlic and garlic salt and mix well until smooth. And set aside
10. Add Italian seasoning and then red pepper flakes to a jar of marinara sauce and stir well. Set aside
11. Now add a layer of sliced zucchini to the baking dish.

12. Spread ¼ cup of the cheese mixture over the zucchini.
13. Afterward, add ¼ of the sausage over the cheese. Add a layer of sauce over the sausage
14. Repeat this layering processes, over and over until all of the ingredients are used, and end with a layer of sauce.
15. Now add the remaining mozzarella cheese and sprinkle with parmesan
16. Cover the dish with tin foil and bake for 30 minutes
17. After 30 minutes, remove a foil and bake for another 15 minutes until golden brown
18. Remove from oven, and then allow it to cool down for 5 minutes before serving
19. Sprinkle with fresh basil

DINNER: Roasted Chicken Stacks

Ingredients

- Chicken breasts
- or chicken breast cutlets 5 small
- Savoy cabbage 1 head
- Coconut flour 3 tbsp.
- Prosciutto 5 slices
- Bone broth ½ cup
- Italian herb blend 2 tbsp
- Avocado oil ¼ cup
- Black pepper 1 tbsp
- Salt 2 tbsp or more to taste

Instructions

1. Preheat the oven to 400°F
2. Put the chicken breasts, salt & pepper, herbs * coconut flour in a large plastic bag.
3. Shake the bag to evenly mix all ingredients and coat the chicken
4. Drizzle a tablespoon of oil on a sheet pan
5. Shred the savoy cabbage finely
6. Place five even piles of cabbage on the sheet pan and sprinkle with some salt, and drizzle with a little oil
7. Place a chicken breast over each pile
8. Top each of chicken breast with a slice of prosciutto and drizzle with the remaining oil
9. Place the sheet pan into the oven and bake for 30 minutes
10. Pour the broth from the sheet pan and bake for another 10 minutes
11. Remove from the oven and serve hot

DAY 7

Breakfast: Creamy Scrambled Eggs
Ingredients

- Eggs 8 large
- Heavy cream 4 tbsp
- Grass-fed butter 8 tbsp
- Shredded Cheddar Cheese 2 oz.
- Black pepper to taste
- Salt to taste
- Chopped chives

Instructions

1. In the large skillet, over medium low heat, warm the butter until it melts and starts to bubble
2. While the butter is melting, in the mixing bowl, whisk together the eggs, cream, salt & pepper until creamy and smooth
3. Now pour the mix into the heated skillet
4. Spread cheese over the top and let it sit in the skillet for approximately one minute or until the eggs become opaque around the edges
5. Using a silicone spatula, fold the eggs in towards the center
6. Continue "scrambling" the eggs this way, mixing the melted cheese into the center
7. When eggs are cooked to the desired firmness and the cheese is well combined with it, sprinkle with freshly chopped chives
8. Serve hot

LUNCH: Herbed Balsamic Chicken

Ingredients

- Boneless skinless chicken thighs 1 pounds
- Minced fresh basil 1 tbsp
- Minced fresh chives 1 tbsp
- Minced garlic clove 1 large
- Balsamic vinegar ½ cup
- Virgin olive oil 3 tbsp
- Grated lemon peel 2 tbsp
- Salt ¾ tbsp
- Pepper ¼ tbsp

Instructions

1. In a mixing bowl, add all ingredients (excluding the chicken) and whisk it well
2. Now toss the chicken in the mixture adding a ⅓ cup of the vinegar mixture
3. Let the chicken stand for 10 minutes
4. Cook the chicken, covered, over medium heat, until the thermometer reaches a temperature of 170°F inside the meat – this should take about 6 to 8 minutes on each side
5. When done, remove and drizzle the chicken with the remaining vinegar mixture before serving.

DINNER: Keto Meatball

Ingredients
Meatball:

- Ground beef 1 pounds
- Egg 1 large
- Shredded mozzarella ½ cup
- Minced garlic 1 clove
- Freshly chopped parsley 2 tbsp
- Freshly grated Parmesan ¼ cup
- Kosher salt 1 tbsp
- Freshly ground black pepper ½ tsp.
- Extra-virgin olive oil 2 tbsp.

Sauce:

- Crushed tomatoes 1 can
- Chopped onion 1 medium
- Minced garlic 2 cloves
- Dried oregano 1 tsp.

- Kosher salt
- Freshly ground black pepper

Instructions

1. In the large mixing bowl, combine the beef, garlic, mozzarella, Parmesan and parsley, eggs, salt & pepper.
2. Mix well and roll the mixture into 16 meatballs
3. Place a large skillet over medium heat and add oil.
4. When oil is hot, add meatballs and cook turning occasionally, until golden brown all around. This should take about ten minutes.
5. Remove meatballs from a skillet and place on a paper towel-lined plate
6. Add onions to the same skillet and cook for 5 minutes or until soft
7. Add some garlic and cook for one minute more until fragrant
8. Now add tomatoes and oregano and season with salt & pepper
9. Add the meatballs back into the skillet.
10. Cover and simmer until the sauce thickens, around 15 minutes.
11. Garnish with Parmesan and serve hot.

~

CONCLUSION

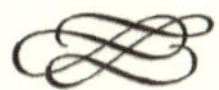

It is hard to write a conclusion for something that is absolutely known as a new beginning. Once you start on the ketogenic lifestyle, you never conclude your membership. You go away, and you come back again.

Doing the keto is much easier than people think, and sometimes much harder than you expect. It is often not the diet or the lifestyle that is really hard. The hardest part is often taking leave of your life – as you know it, with all of its comfort foods and sweets and treats and food memories. Taking leave of this comfort zone is the hard part.

You have to be tired of your lethargic and fat and perpetually lazy existence to really walk away. Overindulgence over the holidays makes for a natural start, but when you're ready, go.

Once you are off, the rest will come easily. The most important thing is to educate yourself properly. You have to follow the right path. Many authors and pundits mislead readers so badly that they end up following strange diets they call keto, which is not.

This book is cutting edge and well informed. Start here.